Cancer Reversal Diet Cookbook

The Ultimate Cardiologist Recommendation Cancer Meal Plan For Old People

28 Days Meal Planner

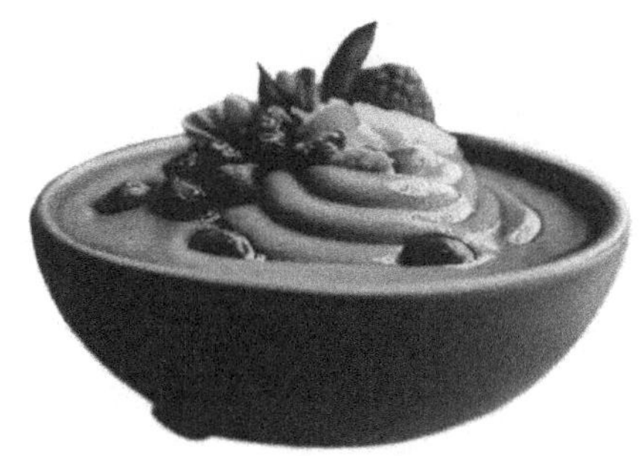

By

Steve Bell

Table of content

Introduction

Nancy was 45 when she received a diagnosis with breast cancer.

She was heartbroken but she had no choice but to fight the disease. She had surgical procedures, chemotherapy, and radiation treatment.

Nancy was told after her treatment that she had a 50% probability of recurrence. She was terrified, but she had no choice but to do all possible to prevent the cancer from returning.

She started researching about the relationship between nutrition and cancer. She discovered that a diet high in fruits, veggies, and whole grains could help prevent and even reverse cancer.

One day, Nancy was surfing through a facebook group when she found a book called "Cancer Reversal Diet Cookbook" by Steve Bell. She had never heard of Steve Bell before, but the title of the book piqued her interest. She started reading the book and was instantly intrigued by the science-backed facts on the connection between diet and cancer.

Nancy decided to implement the diet approach that was mentioned in the book. She began eating more fruits and vegetables, as well as whole grains. She also avoided processed foods, sugary beverages, and red meat.

Within a few months, Nancy started to feel better. Her energy levels rose, and she began to lose weight. Her doctor was delighted with her improvement, and she had regular checkups.

Nancy was cancer-free after a few years. She was thankful for the dietary changes she had made. She was aware that her diet had aided her recovery.

Nancy became an advocate for this book right from the day she got result and improvement in her life. She shared her story with others who are facing cancer on her facebook friend list and also got her coworker a copy of this book to help her reverse the progressing cancer she's suffering from.

Her story shows that there are things you can do to improve your chances of beating the disease.

A healthy diet is one of the most important things you can do to protect your health and fight cancer.

You can get a copy of this gem for the sake of your health and reverse your cancer, and also with the information in this book you can achieve a healthy lifestyle that kicks against cancer.

A diagnosis of cancer can be one of life's hardest difficult and upsetting events, both for the person diagnosed and those closest to them. While medical therapies such as chemotherapy, radiation, and surgery are important in the fight against cancer, there is growing acknowledgment of the importance of diet and nutrition in helping the body's fight against this powerful disease.

The Cancer Diet is not an adequate treatment for cancer, instead serving as a supplement to standard medical therapy. It entails adopting deliberate and informed food choices in order to offer critical nutrients, enhance general health, and maximise your body's capacity to defend itself. This approach recognises the important interplay between nutrition, the immune system, and cellular health, providing people seeking ways to make a difference to their health during their cancer journey with a sense of empowerment.

This comprehensive resource compiles the most recent studies and insights into the role of nutrition in cancer prevention, treatment, and recovery. This cookbook seeks to provide a wealth of knowledge and a wide assortment of tasty, cancer-friendly recipes to nourish and thrill the palate, from comprehending the triggers and risk factors of cancer to investigating the function of certain foods and dietary patterns.

Keep in mind that this is not a solo adventure.

Consult with healthcare specialists, enlist the help of loved ones, and use this cookbook as a resource to improve your general well-being and quality of life during this difficult time.

Let us go on this journey of feeding and healing together, arming ourselves with knowledge and embracing the Cancer Diet's potential as a complementing tool in our battle against cancer.

Chapter 1

Breakfast Delights

Berry Blast Smoothie Bowl

Ingredients:

- 1 ripe banana

- 1 full cup of berry mixture (strawberries, blueberries, and raspberries)

- A half-cup of spinach leaves

- 1/2 cup almond milk that is unsweetened

- Chia seeds, 2 teaspoons

- Kiwi slices, coconut shavings, and pumpkin seeds as toppings

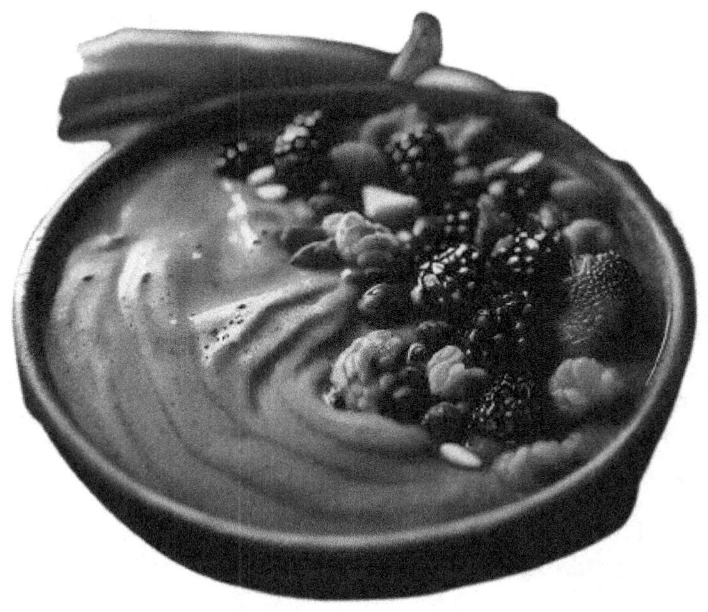

Instructions:

- Blend the berries, banana, spinach, and almond milk until thoroughly combined.

- Add chia seeds, kiwi slices, coconut, and pumpkin seeds to the smoothie's bowl after you've poured it in.

Quinoa Porridge for Breakfast

Ingredients:

- 1 cup unsweetened coconut milk

- 1/2 cup rinsed quinoa

- 1/2 teaspoon cinnamon, ground

- 1 tablespoon maple syrup or honey

- For the topping, use fresh berries and chopped almonds.

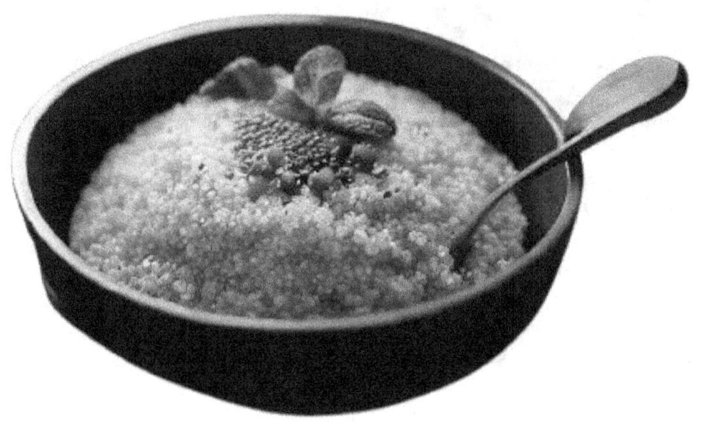

Instructions:

- Combine the quinoa, coconut milk, and cinnamon in a saucepan. When the quinoa is ready, simmer it for a while after turning down the heat.

- Add the sweet maple syrup or just honey then stir.

- Serve the quinoa porridge topped with chopped almonds and fresh berries.

Avocado and Tomato Toast:

Ingredients:

- 1 ripe avocado, mashed

- 2 pieces of whole grain bread

- 1 sliced medium tomato

- Fresh basil leaves

 - garnish with black pepper and salt

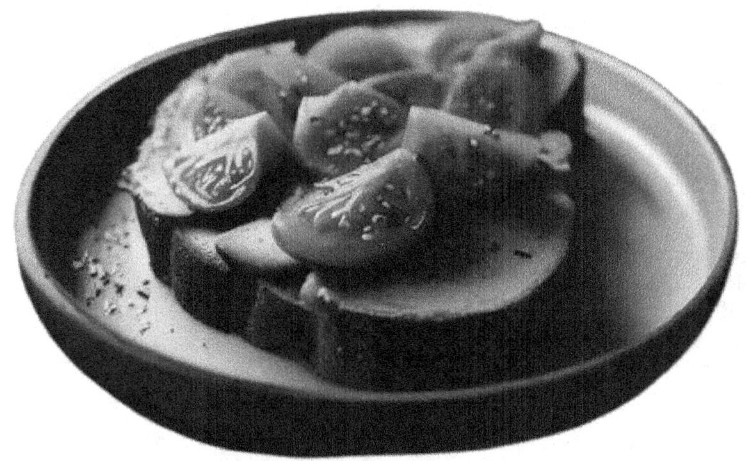

Instructions:

- Spread the mashed avocado on the toast slices according per the instructions.

- Add tomato slices and fresh basil leaves as garnish.

- Add some sea salt and black pepper for seasoning.

Vegetable Omelette:

Ingredients:

- 3 big eggs

- 2 teaspoons of chopped, multicoloured bell peppers

- 1 tablespoon chopped fresh herbs (parsley, basil, or chives)

- 2 tablespoons diced tomatoes

- 2 tablespoons chopped spinach

- To taste-added salt and pepper

- 1 teaspoon olive oil

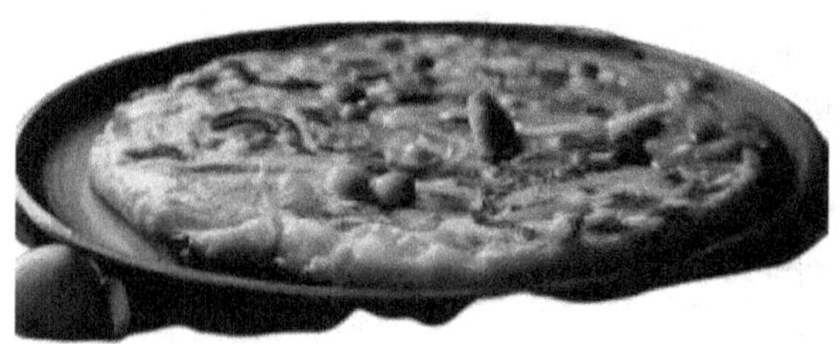

Instructions:

- combine the eggs, bell peppers, tomatoes, spinach, and fresh herbs in a bowl.

- Add salt and pepper to taste.

- In a nonstick pan, warm up the olive oil over medium heat.

- When the omelette is set, pour the egg mixture into the skillet.

- Serve the omelette folded in half.

Mango with Chia Seed Pudding

Ingredients:

- 1-fourth cup of chia seeds

- Unsweetened coconut milk, 1 cup

- 1 tablespoon agave nectar or honey

- 1 sliced ripe mango

- Toasted coconut flakes for decoration

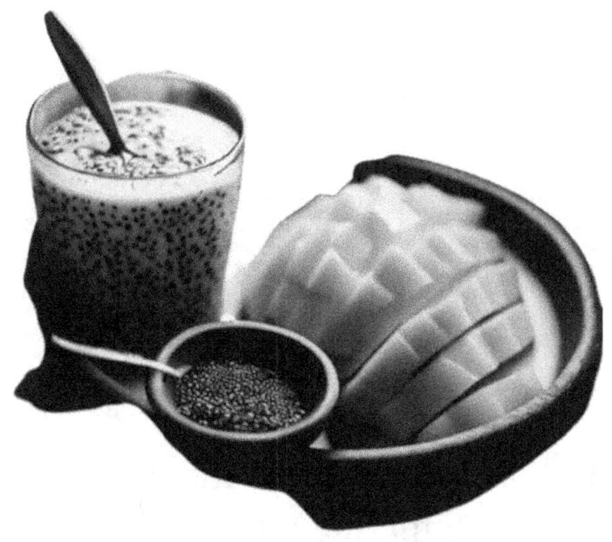

Instructions:

- Chia seeds, coconut milk, and honey or agave syrup should be combined in a bowl. Stir well, then chill for at least two hours or overnight.

- Before serving, top the chia seed pudding with toasted coconut flakes and chopped mango.

Buckwheat pancakes with berries:

Ingredients:

- 1 cup buckwheat flour,

- 1 teaspoon baking powder

- 1 cup of unsweetened almond milk,

- 1 tablespoon of honey or maple syrup, and 1 large egg.

- Fresh berries as a garnish

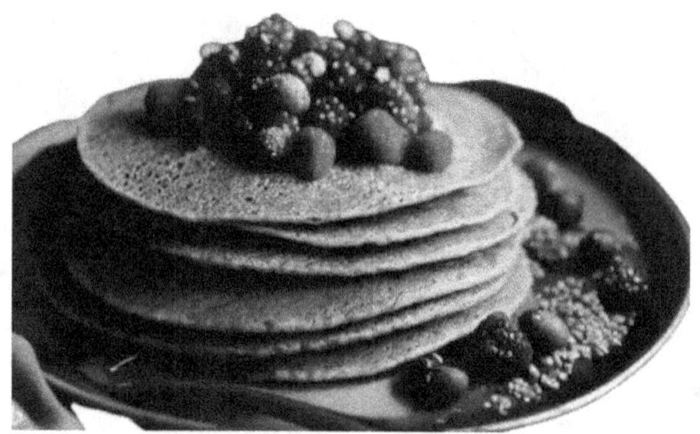

Instructions:

- Buckwheat flour, baking powder, honey or maple syrup, almond milk, and egg should all be combined in a mixing dish and beaten until smooth.

- Pour the pancake batter onto a nonstick skillet that has been heated over medium heat to create tiny pancakes.

- Cook until surface bubbles appear, then turn and continue to cook the other side until golden.

- Put fresh berries on top of the pancakes before serving.

Coconut Yoghurt Parfait:

Ingredients:

- One cup of plain coconut yoghurt

- Half a cup of homemade granola with nuts and seeds

- 1/2 cup of fresh berries blended in.

- 1 tablespoon agave nectar or honey

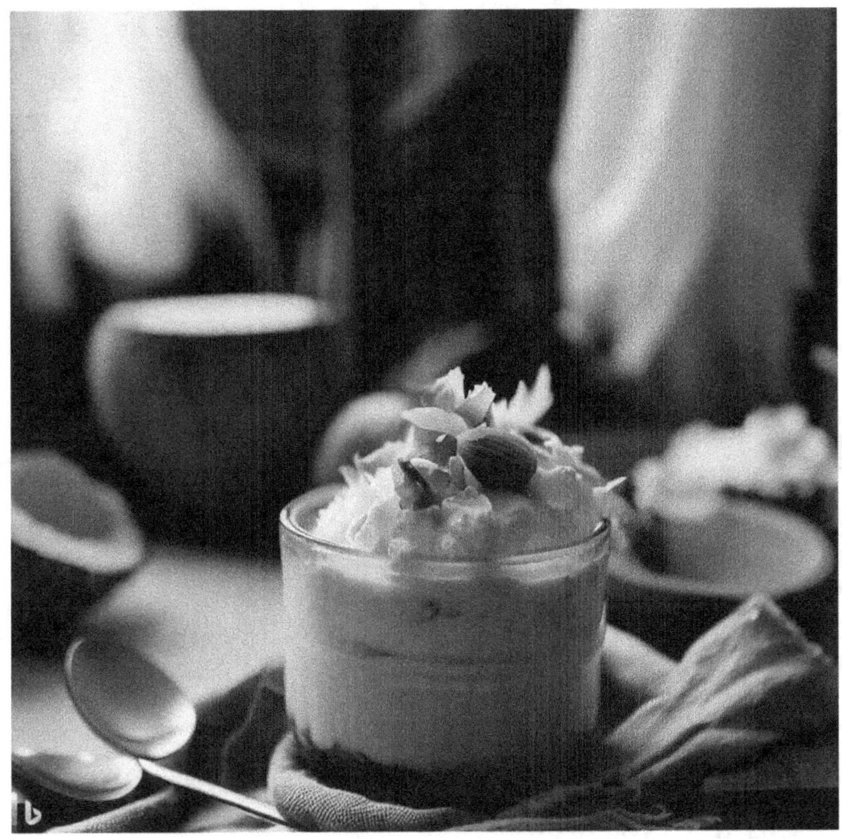

Instructions:

- Layer coconut yoghurt, granola, and fresh berries in a glass or bowl.

- To add more sweetness, drizzle honey or agave syrup over top.

Green Breakfast Smoothie

Ingredients:

- 1 cup almond milk without sugar; 1 ripe banana.

- One cup of fresh spinach leaves

- One teaspoon of almond butter

- A optional 1/2 teaspoon of matcha powder

- Ice cubes, if desired

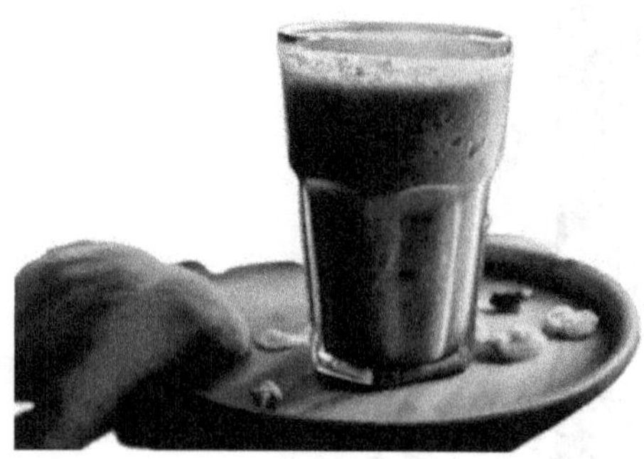

Instructions:

- Blend the following ingredients until smooth: almond milk, banana, spinach, almond butter, and matcha powder.

- To make the smoothie colder, if required, add ice cubes.

Buckwheat Breakfast Bowl

Ingredients:

- 1/4 cup sliced strawberries and

- 1/2 cup cooked buckwheat groats

- One-fourth cup blueberries

- 1 teaspoon finely chopped walnuts

- 1 teaspoon honey or maple syrup

- 1 tablespoon ground flaxseed

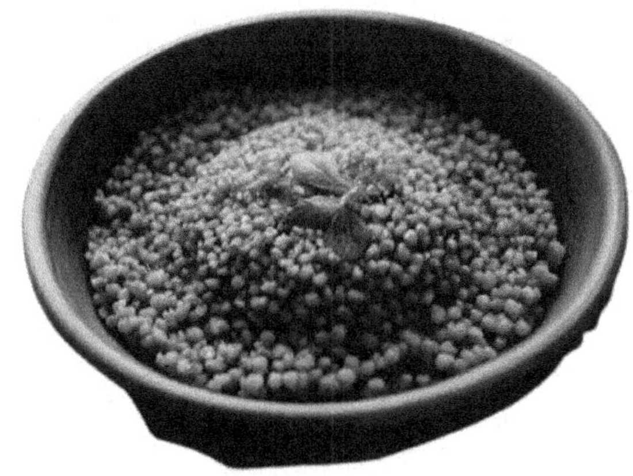

Instructions:

- Prepared buckwheat groats, strawberries, blueberries, chopped walnuts, and ground flaxseed should be combined in a bowl.

- Pour some honey or maple syrup on top for a hint of sweetness.

Turmeric Chai Oatmeal

Ingredients:

- 2 cups of water or plain almond milk

- 1/2 teaspoon each of crushed turmeric and ground cinnamon

- 1 cup of rolled oats

- A dash of black pepper and ground ginger

- 1 tablespoon maple syrup or honey

- Sliced banana and chopped nuts as topping

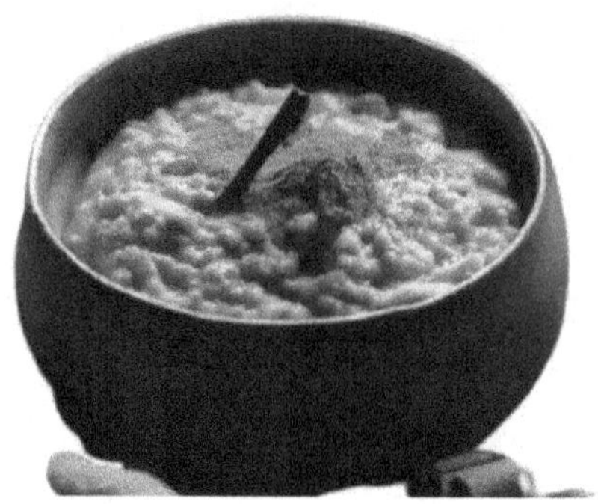

Instructions:

- Oats, water or almond milk, turmeric, cinnamon, ginger, and black pepper should all cook together in a pot.

- Cook the oats until they are soft and creamy.

- Add honey or sweet maple syrup and stir.

- Before serving, garnish with sliced banana and chopped almonds.

These breakfast recipes offer a variety of nutrient-dense choices for individuals following a cancer diet and are created to be both healthy and delightful. Enjoy these healthy breakfasts, and may they help you feel better overall as you battle cancer.

Chapter 2

Lunch Recipes

Quinoa and Roasted Vegetable Salad

Ingredients:

- 1 cup cooked quinoa

- A variety of roasted veggies, including cherry tomatoes, zucchini, and bell peppers

- 1/4 cup crumbled feta cheese (optional)

- Handful of baby spinach leaves

- Lemon-tahini dressing (1 tablespoon tahini, 1 tablespoon lemon juice, 1 tablespoon water, salt, and pepper to taste)

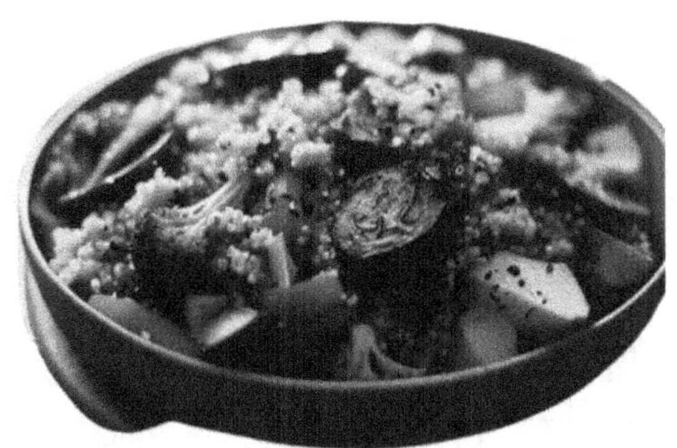

Instructions:

- In a large bowl, combine cooked quinoa, roasted vegetables, feta cheese, and baby spinach.

- Drizzle with lemon-tahini dressing and toss to coat.

Grilled Chicken and Avocado Wrap

Ingredients:

- Grilled chicken breast slices

- Sliced avocado

- Sliced cucumber

- Shredded carrots

- Whole-grain wrap or collard green leaves

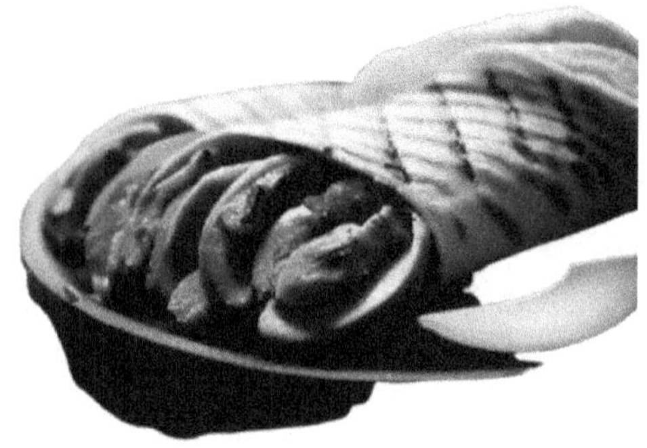

Instructions:

- Lay the wrap or collard green leaves flat and layer with grilled chicken, avocado, cucumber, and shredded carrots.

- Roll up tightly and cut into slices if using a wrap.

Lentil and Vegetable Soup

Ingredients:

- 1 cup cooked lentils

- Assorted vegetables (carrots, celery, onions, tomatoes)

- 4 cups vegetable broth

- 1 teaspoon dried thyme

- Salt and pepper to taste

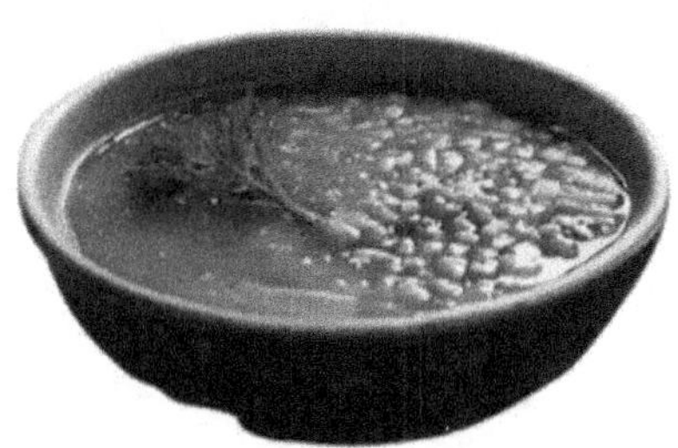

Instructions:

- In a pot, sauté vegetables until softened.

- Add cooked lentils, vegetable broth, dried thyme, salt, and pepper.

- Simmer until the flavors meld together.

Sautéed Salmon with Asparagus and Quinoa
Ingredients:

- Salmon fillet

- Fresh asparagus spears

- 1 cup cooked quinoa

- Lemon slices

- Fresh dill (optional)

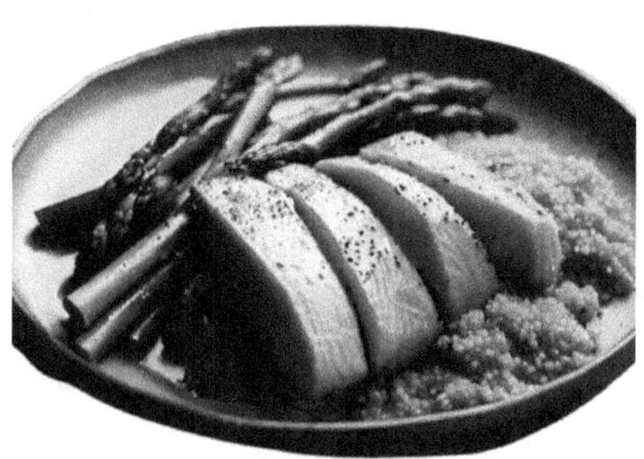

Instructions:

- Sauté the salmon fillet and asparagus spears until cooked through.

- Serve over a bed of quinoa and garnish with lemon slices and fresh dill.

Chickpea and Avocado Salad

Ingredients:

- 1 can chickpeas (drained and rinsed)

- 1 ripe avocado, diced

- Cherry tomatoes, halved

- Chopped cucumber

- Fresh parsley leaves

- Lemon-olive oil dressing (1 tablespoon olive oil, 1 tablespoon lemon juice, salt, and pepper to taste)

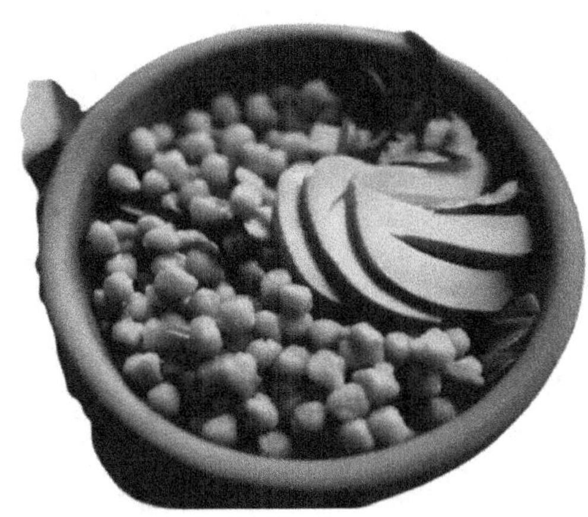

Instructions:

- In a bowl, combine chickpeas, diced avocado, cherry tomatoes, chopped cucumber, and fresh parsley.

- Drizzle with lemon-olive oil dressing and toss gently.

Roasted Vegetable Quiche

Ingredients:

- Whole-grain pie crust (store-bought or homemade)

- Assorted roasted vegetables (broccoli, cauliflower, red onions)

- 4 large eggs

- 1/2 cup unsweetened almond milk

- Salt, pepper, and dried herbs to taste

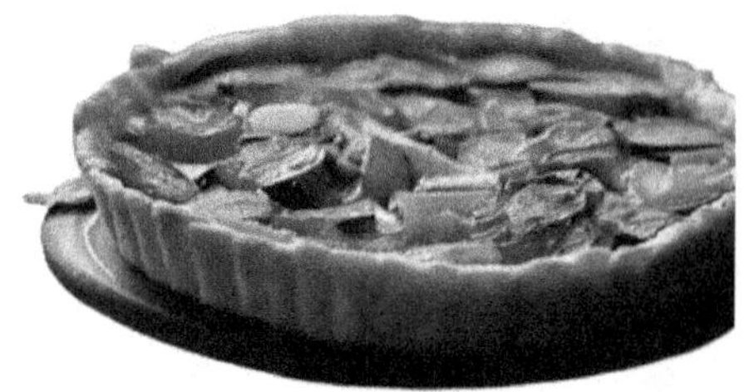

Instructions:

- Preheat the oven according to the pie crust instructions.

- Layer the roasted vegetables in the pie crust.

- In a separate bowl, whisk together eggs, almond milk, salt, pepper, and dried herbs.

- Spread the egg blend over the pie crust's vegetables.

- Bake until the quiche is set and golden brown.

Cucumber and Avocado Gazpacho

Ingredients:

- 2 cucumbers, peeled and diced

- 1 ripe avocado, peeled and pitted

- 1 cup plain Greek yogurt

- 1 tablespoon lime juice

- Handful of fresh cilantro

- Salt and pepper to taste

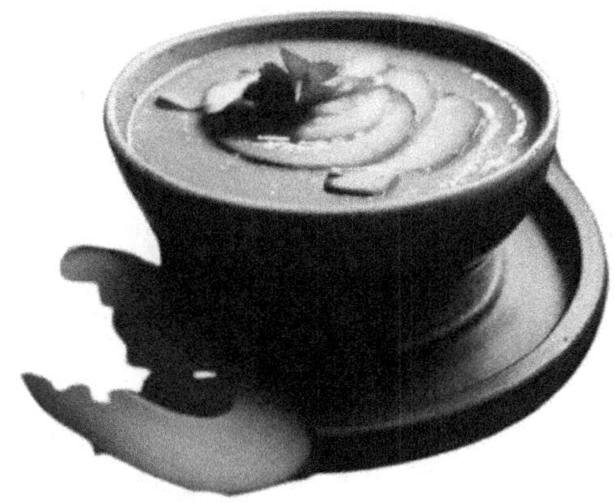

Instructions:

- In a blender, combine cucumbers, avocado, Greek yogurt, lime juice, and cilantro.

- Blend until smooth, adding water if needed to reach the desired consistency.

- Before serving, sprinkle the dish with pepper and salt and place in the refrigerator.

Spinach and Mushroom Quinoa Bowl

Ingredients:

- 1 cup cooked quinoa

- Sautéed spinach and mushrooms

- Toasted pine nuts

- Crumbled goat cheese (optional)

- Balsamic vinaigrette dressing (1 tablespoon balsamic vinegar, 1 tablespoon olive oil, 1 teaspoon Dijon mustard, salt, and pepper to taste)

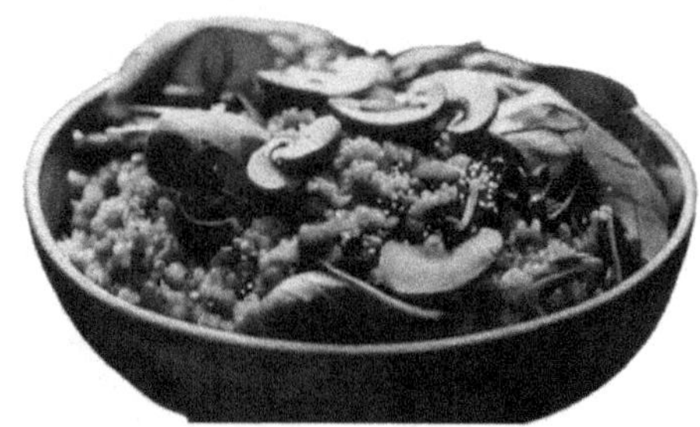

Instructions:

- In a bowl, combine cooked quinoa, sautéed spinach and mushrooms, toasted pine nuts, and crumbled goat cheese.

- Drizzle with balsamic vinaigrette dressing and toss to combine.

Tuna and White Bean Salad

Ingredients:

- Canned tuna (packed in water), drained

- 1 can white beans (cannellini or navy), drained and rinsed

- Sliced red onions

- Sliced bell peppers (assorted colors)

- Fresh basil leaves

- Lemon-Dijon dressing (1 tablespoon lemon juice, 1 tablespoon olive oil, 1 teaspoon Dijon mustard, salt, and pepper to taste)

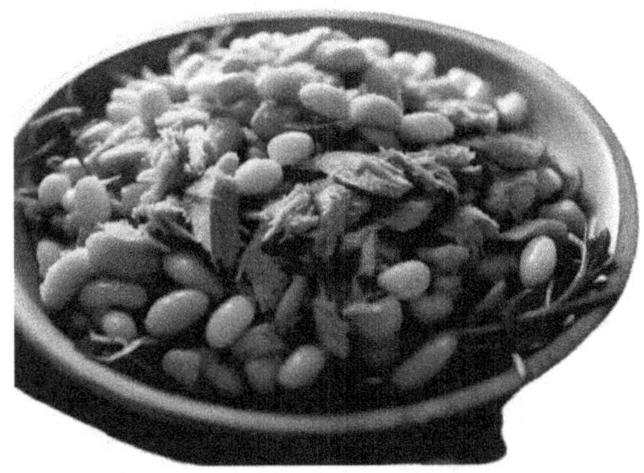

Instructions:

- In a bowl, combine canned tuna, white beans, sliced red onions, bell peppers, and fresh basil.

- Drizzle with lemon-Dijon dressing and toss gently.

Stuffed Bell Peppers with Quinoa and Black Beans

Ingredients:

- Bell peppers (assorted colors), halved and seeded

- 1 cup cooked quinoa

- 1 can black beans, drained and rinsed

- Sliced cherry tomatoes

- Fresh cilantro leaves

- Avocado slices

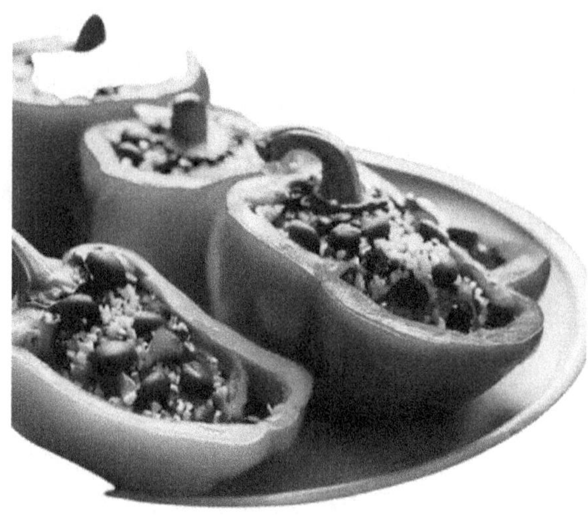

Instructions:

- Preheat the oven to 375°F (190°C).

- In a bowl, mix cooked quinoa, black beans, sliced cherry tomatoes, and fresh cilantro.

- Stuff the halved bell peppers with the quinoa mixture.

- Bake in the oven for about 20-25 minutes or until the peppers are tender.

- Serve with avocado slices on top.

These lunch recipes are designed to be both delicious and nutritious, providing a variety of cancer-fighting ingredients while ensuring a satisfying meal. Enjoy these wholesome lunches and may they contribute to your overall well-being during your cancer journey.

Chapter 3

Dinner Recipes

Baked Lemon-Herb Salmon with Quinoa

Ingredients:

- Salmon fillets

- Lemon slices

- Fresh herbs (rosemary, thyme, or dill)

- 1 cup cooked quinoa

- Steamed broccoli or asparagus

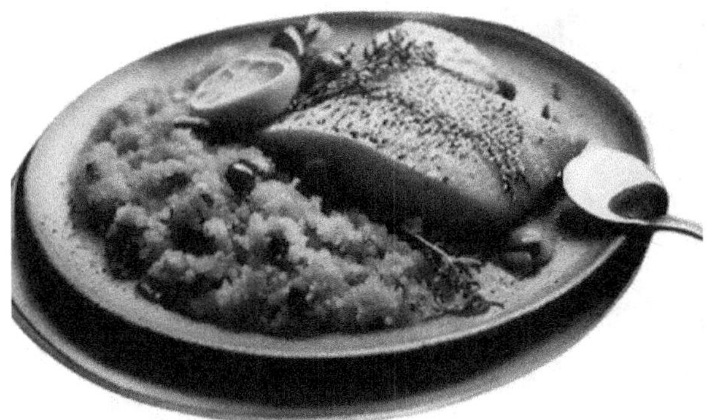

Instructions:

- Preheat the oven to 375°F (190°C).

- Place the salmon fillets on a baking sheet and top each with lemon slices and fresh herbs.

- Bake the salmon in the oven for 15 to 20 minutes, or until it is done.

- Serve with cooked quinoa and steamed broccoli or asparagus.

Brown Rice Stir-Fry with Tofu and Vegetables

Ingredients:

- Firm tofu, cubed

- Assorted vegetables (bell peppers, broccoli, snap peas, carrots)

- 1 cup cooked brown rice

- Stir-fry sauce (1 tablespoon soy sauce, 1 tablespoon hoisin sauce, 1 teaspoon sesame oil)

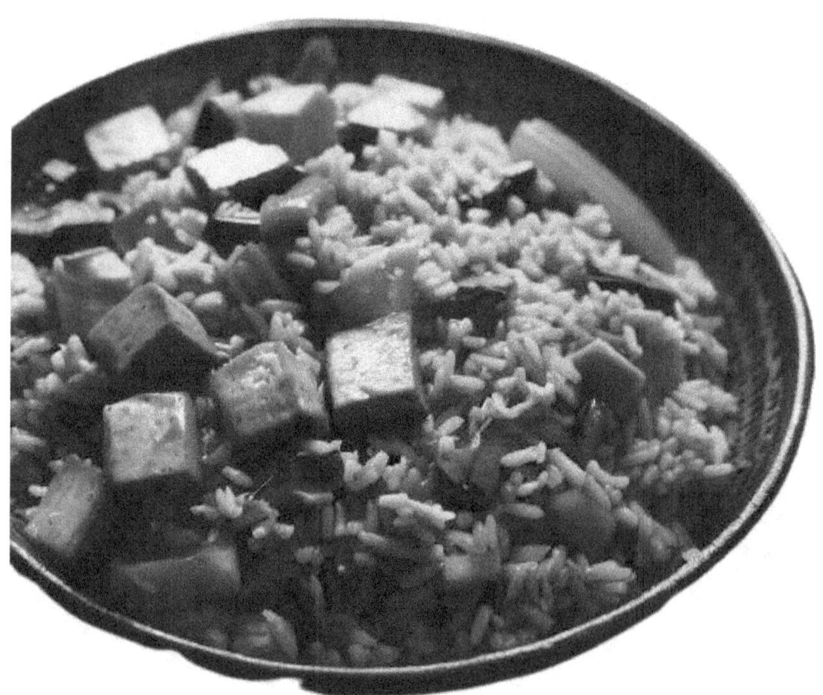

Instructions:

- In a non-stick skillet, sauté tofu and vegetables until lightly browned.

- Add the cooked brown rice and stir-fry sauce, tossing everything together until well combined.

Spaghetti Squash with Tomato and Basil Sauce

Ingredients:

- One spaghetti squash, cut in half and seeded

- Tomato and basil sauce (store-bought or homemade with fresh tomatoes and basil)

- Grated Parmesan cheese (optional)

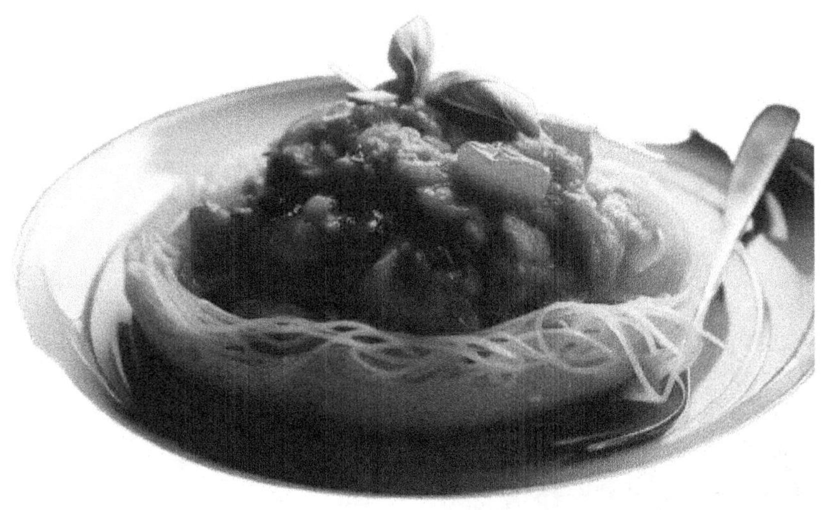

Instructions:

- Preheat the oven to 400°F (200°C).

- Place the spaghetti squash halves, cut-side down, on a baking sheet and bake for about 30-40 minutes or until tender.

- To remove the squash strands, use a fork.

- Top with tomato and basil sauce and sprinkle with grated Parmesan cheese if desired.

Grilled Chicken with Sweet Potato and Brussels Sprouts

Ingredients:

- Grilled chicken breast

- Roasted sweet potato wedges

- Roasted Brussels sprouts

- Seasoning ingredients: garlic, olive oil, pepper and salt.

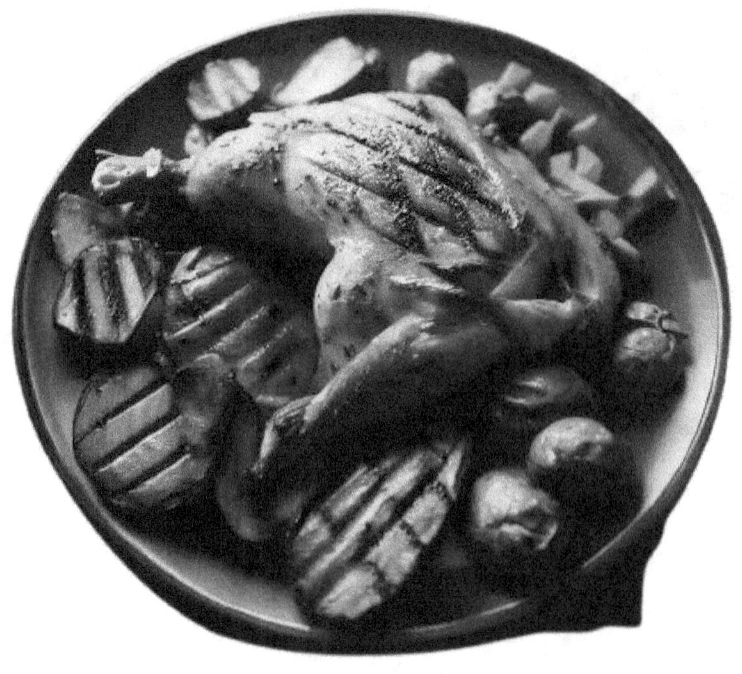

Instructions:

- Season the chicken breast with olive oil, garlic, salt, and pepper, and grill until cooked through.

- Serve with roasted sweet potato wedges and Brussels sprouts.

Veggie Lentil Curry

Ingredients:

- 1 cup cooked lentils

- Assorted vegetables (cauliflower, carrots, peas)

- Coconut milk

- Curry powder or curry paste

- Cooked brown rice or quinoa for serving

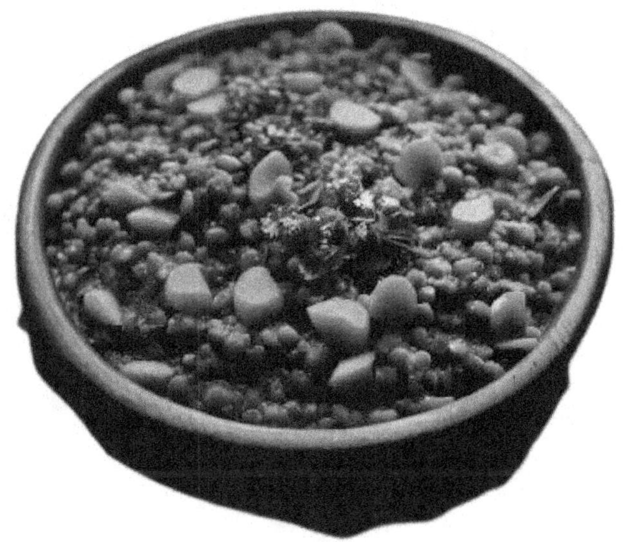

Instructions:

- In a pot, combine cooked lentils, vegetables, coconut milk, and curry powder or paste.

- Simmer for a while to let the flavours mingle and the vegetables become soft.

- Arrange over cooked quinoa or brown rice.

Zucchini Noodles with Pesto and Cherry Tomatoes

Ingredients:

- Zucchini, spiralized into noodles

- Homemade or store-bought basil pesto

- Cherry tomatoes, halved

- Toasted pine nuts

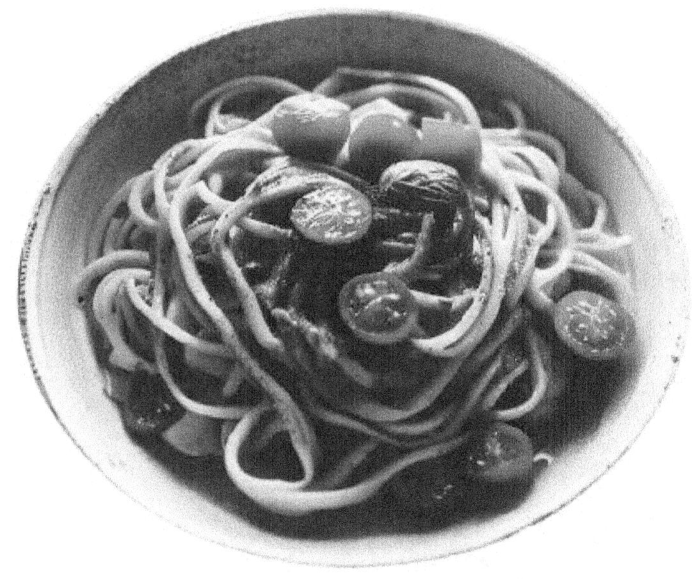

Instructions:

- In a pan, sauté zucchini noodles until tender.

- Toss the zucchini noodles with basil pesto and top with cherry tomatoes and toasted pine nuts.

Grilled Shrimp and Avocado Salad

Ingredients:

- Grilled shrimp

- Mixed greens

- Sliced avocado

- Sliced cucumbers

- Toasted pumpkin seeds

- Lime-cilantro dressing (1 tablespoon lime juice, 1 tablespoon olive oil, fresh cilantro, salt, and pepper to taste)

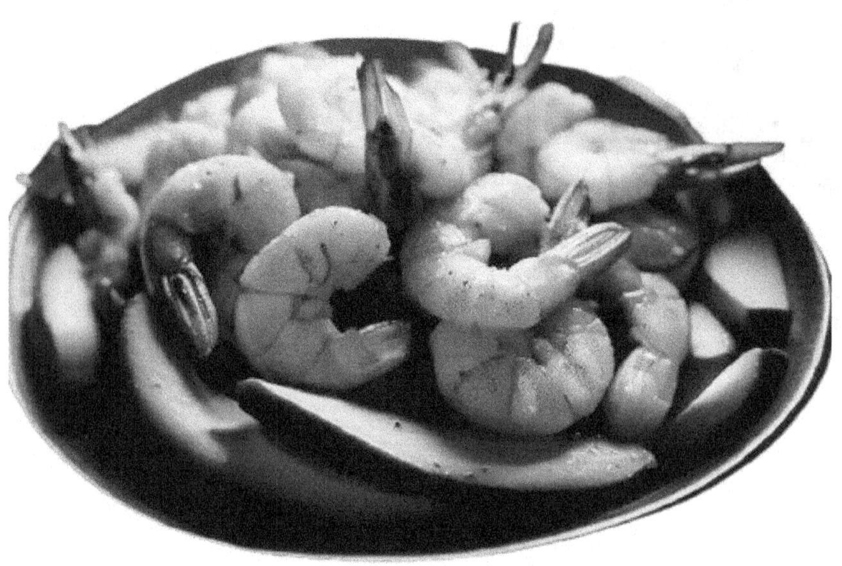

Instructions:

- In a large bowl, combine mixed greens, sliced avocado, sliced cucumbers, and grilled shrimp.

- Drizzle with lime-cilantro dressing and top with toasted pumpkin seeds.

Stuffed Bell Peppers with Quinoa and Chickpeas

Ingredients:

- Bell peppers (assorted colors), halved and seeded

- 1 cup cooked quinoa

- 1 can chickpeas, drained and rinsed

- Diced tomatoes

- Fresh parsley or cilantro

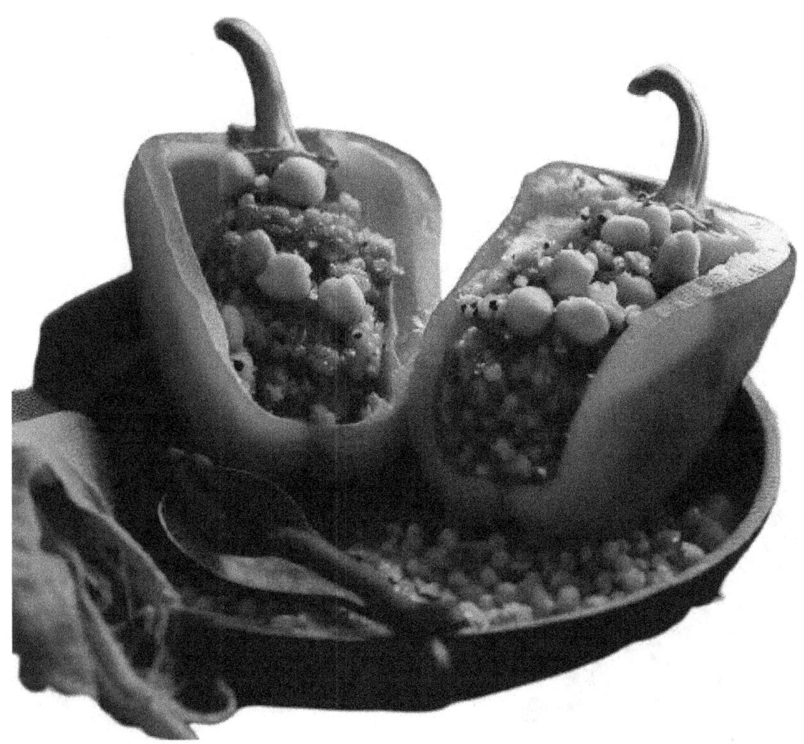

Instructions:

- Preheat the oven to 375°F (190°C).

- In a bowl, mix cooked quinoa, chickpeas, and diced tomatoes.

- Stuff the halved bell peppers with the quinoa-chickpea mixture.

- Bake in the oven for about 20-25 minutes or until the peppers are tender.

- Before serving, garnish with fresh parsley or cilantro.

Baked Cod with Mediterranean Salsa

Ingredients:

- Cod fillets

- Chopped tomatoes

- Chopped cucumbers

- Chopped red onions

- Chopped Kalamata olives

- Chopped fresh parsley

- Lemon juice and olive oil for dressing

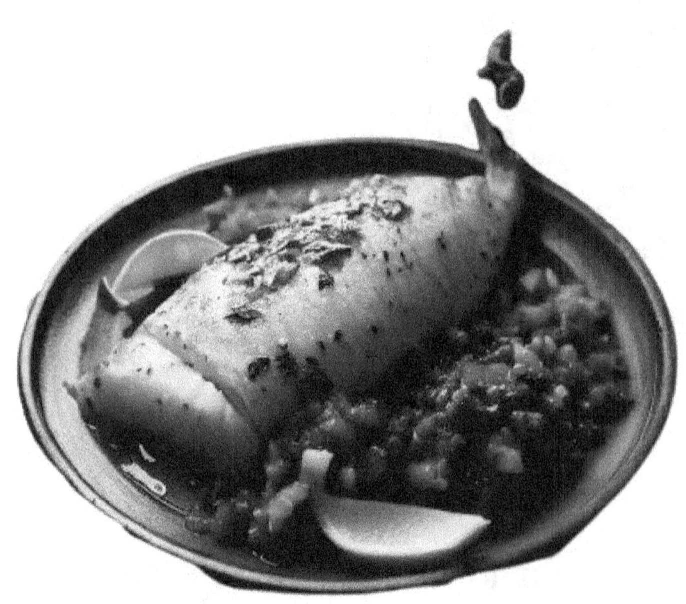

Instructions:

- Preheat the oven to 375°F (190°C).

- Place the cod fillets on a baking sheet and bake until cooked through.

- In a bowl, combine chopped tomatoes, cucumbers, red onions, Kalamata olives, and fresh parsley.

- Drizzle with lemon juice and olive oil to make the Mediterranean salsa.

- Serve the baked cod with the salsa on top.

Vegetable Curry with Turmeric Rice

Ingredients:

- Assorted vegetables (bell peppers, carrots, cauliflower, potatoes)

- Coconut milk

- Curry powder or curry paste

- 1 cup cooked turmeric-infused rice

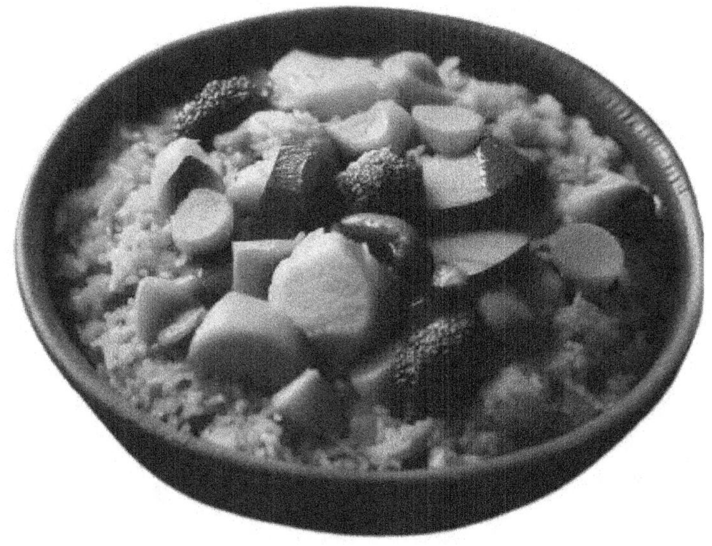

Instructions:

- In a pot, combine the assorted vegetables, coconut milk, and curry powder or paste.

- Simmer for a while to let the flavours mingle and the vegetables become soft

- Serve over cooked turmeric-infused rice.

These dinner recipes are designed to be both delicious and nutritious, providing a variety of cancer-fighting ingredients while ensuring a satisfying and wholesome meal. Enjoy these nourishing dinners and may they contribute to your overall well-being during your cancer journey.

Chapter 4

Snacks and Appetizers for Healing

Baked Sweet Potato Fries

Ingredients:

- Sweet potatoes, cut into thin fries

- 1 tablespoon olive oil

- 1/2 teaspoon paprika

- 1/2 teaspoon garlic powder

- Salt and pepper to taste

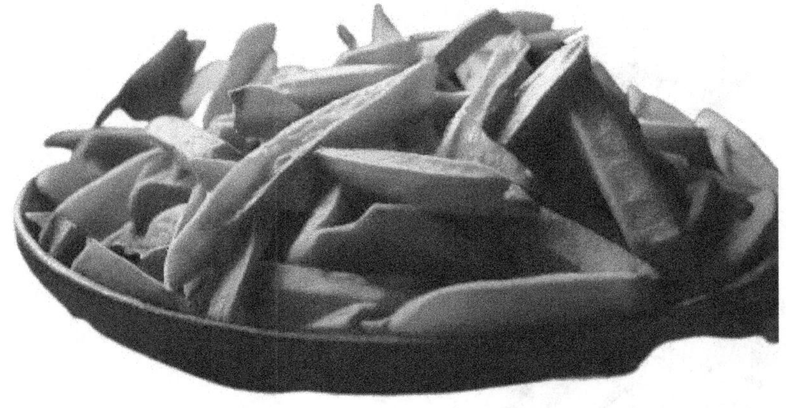

Instructions:

- Preheat the oven to 425°F (220°C).

- In a bowl, toss sweet potato fries with olive oil, paprika, garlic powder, salt, and pepper.

- Spread the fries out on a baking pan in a single layer.

- Bake for about 20-25 minutes or until the fries are crispy and golden brown.

Hummus with Veggie Sticks

Ingredients:

- Homemade or store-bought hummus

- Mixed vegetable sticks (cucumbers, bell peppers, carrots)

- Whole-grain pita wedges

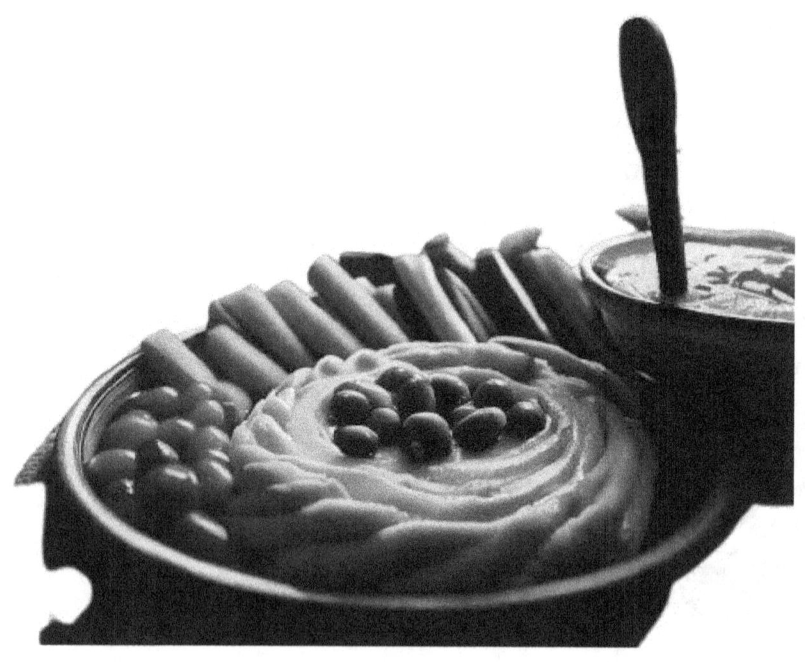

Instructions:

- Serve hummus with vegetable sticks and whole-grain pita wedges for a delicious and nutritious dip.

Guacamole with Homemade Veggie Chips

Ingredients:

- Ripe avocados, mashed

- Diced tomatoes

- Chopped red onions

- Chopped cilantro

- Lime juice, salt, and pepper to taste

- Homemade veggie chips (thinly sliced sweet potatoes or beets)

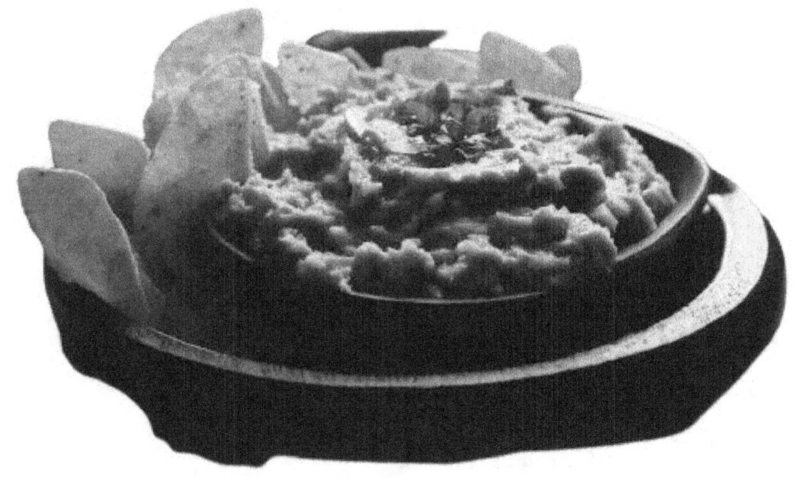

Instructions:

- In a bowl, combine mashed avocados, diced tomatoes, chopped red onions, chopped cilantro, lime juice, salt, and pepper to make guacamole.

- Serve with homemade veggie chips for a flavorful and colorful snack.

Spicy Roasted Chickpeas

Ingredients:

- 1 can chickpeas, drained and rinsed

- 1 tablespoon olive oil

- 1 teaspoon ground cumin

- 1/2 teaspoon smoked paprika

- 1/4 tsp. cayenne pepper (adjust to your own level of spiciness)

- Salt to taste

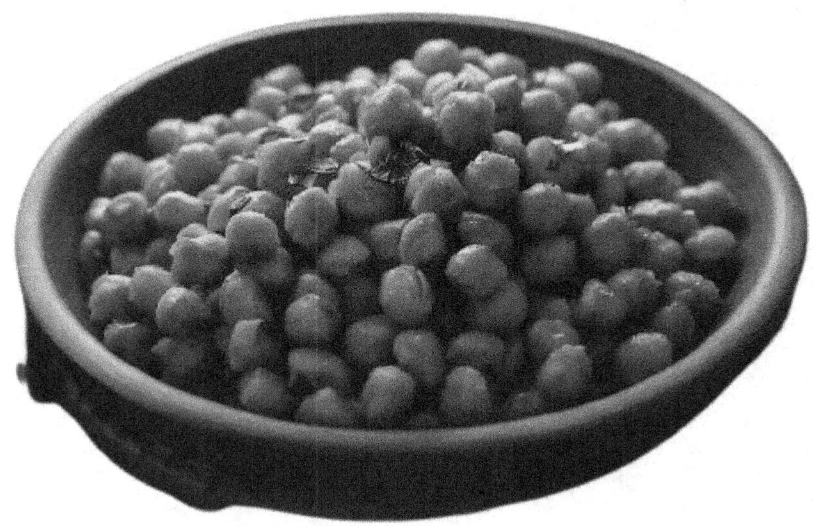

Instructions:

- Preheat the oven to 400°F (200°C).

- In a bowl, toss chickpeas with olive oil, ground cumin, smoked paprika, cayenne pepper, and salt.

- Arrange the chickpeas on a baking sheet in a single layer.

- Roast until crispy for around 25 to 30 minutes.

Berry Chia Seed Pudding Cups

Ingredients:

- 1/4 cup chia seeds

- 1 cup unsweetened almond milk

- 1 tablespoon honey or maple syrup

- Fresh berries (strawberries, blueberries, raspberries)

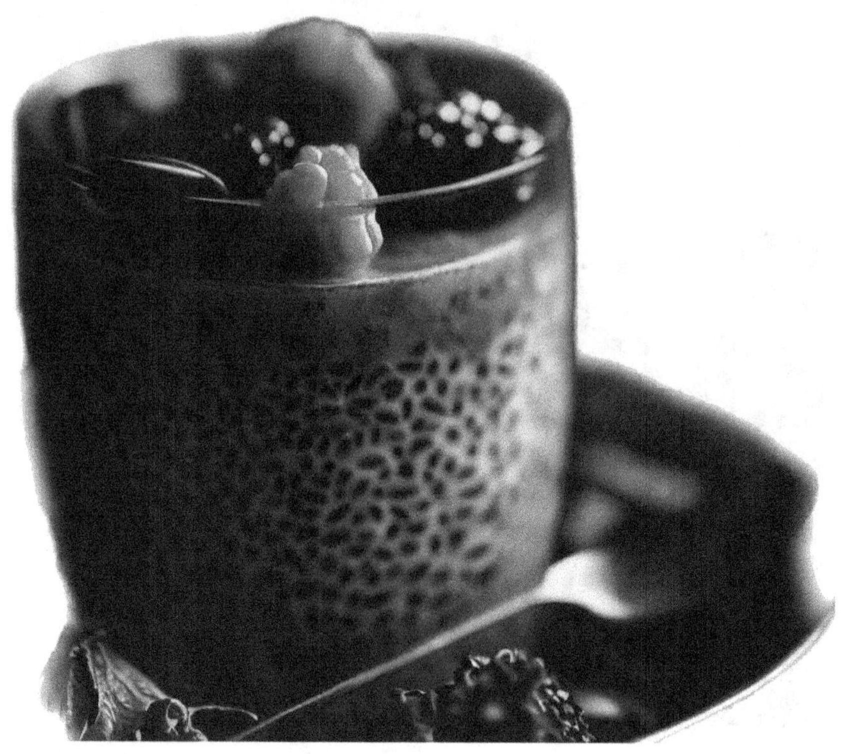

Instructions:

- In a bowl, mix chia seeds, almond milk, and honey or maple syrup. Stir well and refrigerate overnight or for at least 2 hours until the mixture thickens.

- Layer chia seed pudding with fresh berries in small cups for a delightful and nutritious snack.

These snacks and appetizer recipes are not only delicious but also packed with cancer-fighting nutrients. Enjoy these wholesome snacks and appetizers on your cancer journey!

Conclusion

As we reach the final chapter of this Cancer Diet Cookbook, we reflect on the journey we've taken together—a journey of nourishment, knowledge, and empowerment. Throughout these pages, we have explored the powerful connection between nutrition and cancer, recognizing the potential impact of the foods we choose on our bodies' resilience and well-being. While this cookbook cannot provide a cure for cancer, it is a testament to the strength of the human spirit and the transformative power of mindful dietary choices.

We began by delving into the understanding of cancer, its causes, and how certain dietary patterns can contribute to its prevention. Armed with knowledge, we embraced the philosophy that while a cancer diet is not a replacement for medical treatments, it can be an essential complement, supporting the body's natural defenses and fostering an environment conducive to healing.

The heart of this cookbook lies in the carefully curated recipes, each crafted to include cancer-fighting ingredients without compromising on flavor and enjoyment. From vibrant smoothie bowls to hearty main courses, every dish is a celebration of nourishment and a step towards taking control of our health. We have explored creative ways to incorporate a colorful array of fruits, vegetables, whole grains, and plant-based proteins—each ingredient offering its unique benefits.

Throughout this journey, we also acknowledged that each cancer journey is unique, as are the nutritional needs of individuals undergoing various treatments and in different stages of recovery. The meal plans provided were thoughtfully designed to accommodate the specific demands of chemotherapy, radiation therapy, and posttreatment care. We recognized that adapting recipes to personal preferences and dietary restrictions fosters a sense of empowerment in making choices that resonate with individual lifestyles.

Beyond the kitchen, we have emphasized the importance of embracing a holistic approach to health and well-being. Mindful eating practices, regular physical activity, and stress management contribute to the overall healing process. We have sought to inspire a mindset of hope and resilience, recognizing that nourishment extends beyond the plate and into our emotional and mental spheres.

As we close this chapter on the Cancer Diet Cookbook, our hope is that it serves as more than just a collection of recipes. May it be a beacon of hope for those facing the challenges of cancer—a reminder that every meal prepared with love and intention is a gesture of self-care and empowerment. May it inspire individuals on their cancer journey to embrace the potential of a cancer-friendly diet as a partner in their fight for health.

In our collective effort to navigate the complexities of cancer, let us remember that we are not alone. Together, as a community of fighters, survivors, and caregivers, we can lift each other up and forge ahead with courage and determination. With the support of healthcare professionals, the love of family and friends, and the knowledge gained from this cookbook, we embark on a path of nourishment, healing, and hope.

As you continue your journey, remember to remain informed, consult with your healthcare team, and adapt these recipes to your unique needs. Savor each bite, celebrate each small victory, and know that you are making a difference—one nourishing choice at a time.

May this cookbook be a constant companion—a source of inspiration, strength, and a reminder of the profound impact we have on our bodies and lives through the choices we make. Together, let us nourish our bodies, fuel our spirits, and embrace a future filled with health, vitality, and the unwavering hope that lies within us all.

Thank you!!!!

Meal Planner-available in the
paperback version